After Cancer By Lori

Lori Baran

The information found in this book is intended to help and guide you towards healthier choices, but is not intended to replace the services of a qualified medical professional. Seek medical attention, if a health issue is present.

Any mention of an organization, product, service, company, or professional does not imply endorsement by either the author or the publisher. Any adverse effect arising from the use or misuse of the information, from this book, is the sole responsibility of the reader and not that of the author or publisher.

dedication: To Dr. Mark Rosenberg, for your treatment and my life!

To my friends and family, for your unwavering support and love.

To my mom, the late Ann Paul, who's spirit inspires me.

TABLE OF CONTENTS

PREFACE: I am a stage IV metastatic breast cancer survivor. I have had the good fortune of having key people introduced to me, at the right times. I have been asked, numerous times by people that I know, to share what has worked for me. Although these particular methods have worked for me, I do not claim to have a cure for cancer, nor do I recommend that anyone adopt this protocol on their own. Please consult and work closely with a physician. This book is a collection of my thoughts and feelings, and is in no way meant to give medical advice to anyone. Find an alternative doctor, who you trust with your life, and begin your healing process.

Good Luck!

AFTER CANCER

For four years, it has been take one step forward, then two backwards. It was month after month of looking in the mirror and hating what I was seeing. I kept looking within, to find the old me, which was longing to come out. Where should I begin and where was I going? Is the "old me" still there? Would cancer control me or would I control the cancer? I couldn't help but dream about the past when I had a good figure and was full of life and energy. Could a future exist, where I could be *that* happy again? I had to find the girl from "back then", in that "happy place". Until I found her, I knew I could not be whole again.

As I lay here, in the hyperbaric oxygen chamber, I have plenty of time to reflect on my journey. Less than one year ago, a very good friend of mine, from my past, asked me two questions:"Did your life turn out like you thought it would?" and "Are you happy?" I knew that with having cancer, gaining lots of weight, having no hair from chemo, and having no job, the answer to both questions was clearly "no"! No one ever thinks that they will get cancer. I certainly didn't and I certainly wasn't happy with the way I felt or looked. But something clicked that day, when I was forced to think about those two questions. I knew that only I had the power to change *"what is"*.

I was soon to find out that my battle with cancer was not over, following my bilateral mastectomy. That was definitely the lowest point in my life. I had lost hope. When you lose hope, you lose everything….your will to live and your self-esteem. You just get tired of it all and give up. That is when you die! I did know one thing. I was not ready to die, so I decided it was time to fight back!

***

LESSONS LEARNED

I do believe that everything happens to us for a reason and that everyone who is brought into our lives has a purpose. And most important of all, we are all in this life to learn lessons. I started to ask myself, "What was my lesson in life to learn?" and "What was my purpose?"

I began to reflect on my past, desperate to find answers to restore my hope. It was a warm summer day, in 1973, when my mother and I were sitting on our front porch, at our house in Dearborn, Michigan. I remember so vividly, as though it were yesterday, my mom telling me that she had uterine cancer. I cried, as my mom explained that she *might* have a year to live, if she has chemo and radiation. She explained to me that she would not be spending her last days debilitated from chemo and radiation, and that she would fight the "big C" her way. My mom, Ann, was 49 years old, at the time. She was diagnosed at about the same time in her life as I was. I can now only imagine how scared she must have been! You really don't know how someone feels until it happens to you! Little did I know that my mom's strength and tenacity would someday save my own life.

My mom never did go back to the oncologist's office, after her hysterectomy and cancer diagnosis.

She attributed her cancer to hormone replacement therapy. She did a lot of reading and research on fighting cancer, holistically. She became a vegetarian, took supplements, and walked on a daily basis. She rarely ever mentioned her cancer again and went on with life, with more hope and determination than I have ever seen. She finally lost her battle with cancer at the age of 81. She exceeded her expected survival time by 32 years! She was the strongest person I have ever known, and I have always felt as though her strength and spirit is with me.

***

MY JOURNEY

My nightmare began, in January of 2008, with a routine mammogram for my physical. This was the first time I was to have a digital mammogram. Several days after the mammogram, came the call from my doctor saying that there were micro-calcifications, within a highly suspicious cluster, in the right breast. A biopsy was needed to exclude malignancy. I had the biopsy done in the middle of February and the results showed ductal carcinoma in-situ. I had breast cancer. The good news, or so I thought, was that it was caught early. The most common treatment is a lumpectomy and radiation. I opted for the bilateral mastectomy. I wanted to take away any and all fear that this cancer would return. I would opt for the drastic route! I also did a lot of research into radiation and wanted to avoid it, at all costs. Especially in the chest area, radiation can cause hardening of the arteries, cancer, and a number of other problems. I have known people who have died from complications of radiation. I was not going to become a statistic, so no radiation for me. I was told that if I had a lumpectomy that I would *have* to have the radiation. I chose to have both breasts removed, not only to look symmetrical, but also why not get some new perky breasts. lol. After all, I may as well get something positive out of this grim situation.

A mutual friend introduced a new friend to me. Kelley had just undergone a bilateral mastectomy with reconstruction. Surprisingly, she not only had the same type of cancer as I did, but she had the same breast surgeon and plastic surgeon! What are the odds of that? Remember when I said that everyone is brought into your life for a reason! I'm just saying!!! Coincidence, I think not. She was totally happy with her decision and the work that was done on her was fabulous! She is an incredibly strong and positive woman! This meeting would seal my decision to have the bilateral mastectomy. It was an easy decision on my part, after meeting Kelley.

The surgery was scheduled for April 16th, 2008. My mom had passed away on April 14th, 3 years prior, and my dad on April 15th, 13 years prior. The date scared me a little bit, but I got a sense of calm that my mom and dad would be watching over me. The reconstruction is done at the same time as the mastectomy, and the expanders are put in to stretch your skin for the implants. It's great because you come out of surgery with cleavage!

Three months after the mastectomy, I had the implants put in. All was well after that, for a while that is. I had to have an implant replaced, due to scar tissue, 15 months after they were put in. Then, two years after the mastectomy, the real nightmare began. I felt a lump under my right arm and went to see my breast surgeon. Chances were slim to none that it was malignant, considering that the three lymph nodes directly in the pathway of the cancer, and removed at the time of the mastectomy, were benign. Then came the call from my breast surgeon, Dr. Linsey Gold, that my axillary lymph node was malignant. How could this be? How could the breast cancer, that was stage I, have gotten through to my lymph nodes? I was devastated! The PET scan on 6/8/10 showed multiple metastatic nodes and three spots on my liver. Surgery was scheduled for the following day. In a grueling 6½ hour surgery, 38 axillary nodes were removed and later pathology would reveal that they were all malignant. Dr. Linsey Gold did a remarkable job, taking care to find and remove all present axillary lymph nodes, while preserving the integrity of my arm.

She is an amazing surgeon! I am so blessed to have had her and the entire team, including Kim Pierson, in the O.R. I know that they were all exhausted after that surgery! Two weeks later, on June 24th, a port was implanted and I began my 4 months of chemotherapy on July 10th.

In the beginning, I was fine. Even though I sat there with everyone else, receiving the chemo, I was still feeling like none of it was real. I was still in denial. So many of the people looked fragile and sick. Many were having multiple side affects from the chemo. I, on the other hand, felt fine. I asked to have my steroids cut back, and had very little, to no nausea. I was hoping to lose some weight. I am always looking for some positive out of a bad situation. Unfortunately, I gained weight. Not what I had wanted, but I needed to stay nutritionally sound.

I had given up all processed food, bottled water, and sugar. I started to walk, and continued to play golf. I was not going to let chemo dictate what I could and couldn't do. It all seemed more real when my hair started to fall out, about a month after the chemo begin. I also lost my eyelashes and eyebrows. There was hair everywhere! It was in the bed, in the shower, and all over the house. I finally asked my husband to shave my head. As I sat on the floor and cried, hair fell all around me. Now I was fat and bald. It doesn't get any worse than that! Looking back in retrospect, that was probably the lowest point of this whole journey. How could I ever be the same? Would I ever be the same?

I was prepared though, for the loss of my golden locks. I had previously gone to *Katie's Spa* in Lapeer, MI. and picked out a wig along with some hat hair. My good friend, Debi, knows the owner, Kim Adams. Again, I cannot repeat this enough. Everyone who is brought into your life has a purpose. Without my friend, Debi, I would not have met Kim when I did. She is an amazing person. Her spa is named after Katie Kirkpatrick-Godwin, a young girl who died of brain cancer, and inspired Kim to create the spa to help cancer patients. It serves as a tribute, to Katie's legacy of helping others. Kim treated me with great respect and dignity. I know that Katie is smiling down upon her, for all that she gives back to cancer patients! Katie's Spa offers several services and products, including wigs, turbans, hats, massages, craniosacral therapy, facials, manicures, pedicures, and waxing. They also have an infrared sauna and a boutique.

My dear friend, Pam, who sat through my surgeries with my husband, also came with me to pick out my wig. I had fun trying on all the different wigs! If you think that "blonds have more fun", then here's your chance! I opted for a wig that looked like my current hairstyle. My good friend, Candy, at *Summerset Salon & Day Spa*, in Flint, MI., colored my real hair to look like the wig, and cut the wig to look like my real hair. When I made the transition to my wig, nobody could tell. Since then, *Summerset Salon & Day Spa*, owned by Candy's daughter, Summer, now carries a full line of wigs, along with being a full service spa. Another great place for pampering!

I felt so blessed to have the support of so many people, and I knew I did not want to give up. I received chemo from July to November. I very rarely felt nauseous and even continued to golf. One of the chemo drugs that I was receiving was light sensitive. Even after applying the 100 SPF sunblock, my skin would be glowing red after 1 minute of sun exposure. My dear husband would hold the umbrella over my head, while I would "putt out". Bless his heart! The whole chemo experience was surreal. I was hooked up to the IV's, going into my port, but I didn't feel like I had cancer. What does cancer feel like? I really didn't feel any different than usual, except that I was scared to death.

I whizzed through chemotherapy and before I knew it, it was over. Having two friends of mine, Bill and Mark, going through chemo at the same time, helped a lot. They were always there for support. I had a PET scan in December and it showed abnormal lymph nodes around my lungs. A mediastinoscopy was performed, by a cardiologist, and biopsies were taken. There was no evidence of primary or metastatic neoplasm within the biopsies. It was probably sarcoidosis. Finally some good news….no cancer! I had my port taken out in January of 2011, against my doctor's wishes. It bothered me constantly, so I wanted it gone. Besides, I was sure I was done with chemo. They would like for you to leave it in for a year, but I couldn't wait another week!

While going through chemo, I changed my eating habits. I cut out all processed foods and started eating organic, most of the time. I felt great when my hair grew back, although it took a lot longer than I would have liked. It was also great to have my eyelashes and eyebrows back. I felt whole once again.

Nine months went by, when I discovered a lump under my left arm. I had a bad feeling this time. I knew in my heart that my cancer was back. I had a biopsy on August 24th, 2011, and the left axillary node came back malignant, as I had expected. Getting the diagnosis, this time, was devastating! I knew that the chemo had failed to kill all of the cancer and probably would not work the second time around, either. I had a chemo drug sensitivity test performed, and the conclusion was that the drugs that I had received should have killed the cancer. So…….now what do I do?????

I started doing some research and my husband and I went to Texas, in search of a treatment that would work. We went in search of HOPE. Unfortunately, we didn't find hope there, only disappointment. The doctors there would inform us that I needed to have all of my lymph nodes removed, in the chest and neck area, and that I should undergo aggressive chemo and radiation. I might have a 2-year survival rate. We came all that way, from Michigan to Texas, to hear that my only hope was 2 years! That was the furthest thing from hope that I have ever known. How could stage I cancer turn into stage IV metastatic cancer? With all the billions of dollars that go into cancer research, shouldn't there be something that could help me? The information that they had given me was totally unacceptable to me. Even though we struck out in Texas, I refused to give up.

Memories of my mom filled my thoughts, and those thoughts consumed my days. I knew that if she could beat cancer, then I could too. I was not a quitter! My family physician, Dr. Longe, had told me that if my cancer was ever to return, that she knew a doctor in Boca Raton, FL., who was doing amazing things to treat cancer patients. He was successful in putting stage IV cancer into remission. His name is one that I will never forget....Dr. Mark Rosenberg. (www.antiagemed.com) A conference call was arranged and we discussed my case. He felt very strongly that he could treat my cancer without surgery, chemo, or radiation. That was music to my ears, *sweet music*. My hope was restored!

He put me on a strict diet and explained how fat cells produce estrogen, and since my cancer was estrogen receptor positive, the fat cells were fueling my cancer. He put me on a ketogenic diet. His plan was for me to lose 60 pounds quickly. The plan also included prescription drugs, supplements, Pleo Alkala, to keep my body alkaline, and hyperbaric oxygen chamber treatments, 3 times a week.

After 4 months of treatments, my MRI came back "markedly improved". My lymph nodes had shrunk and appeared normal! During those four months, I had begun to exercise. I started running and the weight started to fall off. I started to run races (5K's and 8K's) to stay focused. I also joined Weight Watcher's for the support. By the end of 1 year, I had lost 60 pounds and felt terrific!

After 8 months on Dr. Rosenberg's program, my M.R.I. showed perfectly normal lymph nodes. There was no evidence of any cancer. Not only am I cancer free, I feel and look amazing! (At least that is what my friends and family tell me) I am filled with so much gratitude. It was a lot of hard work, but life is so worth it!

I try not to live in a place of fear. It's hard not to think about the cancer coming back. I take one day at a time and know that I have the power to change the outcome, with the help of an amazing doctor! I feel strong and in control of my own destiny, and you can too! We are *all* undeniably powerful people.

At this point, everywhere I go, people ask me how I did it. How did I beat cancer? I know now that my purpose is to help others to find their hope, in an otherwise hopeless situation. I want to make people realize, that we all have the power within us to be strong and survive. I knew that the only other alternative, for me, was death. That, my friends, was never an option. And don't ever let anyone tell you that there is "*no hope*".

I hope that this book has inspired you to *not* give up. One doctor may have given you a death sentence, but that does not mean that you are destined to die. Choose life, get mad, get strong, get educated, seek alternative treatments, make your own decisions, ask questions, and get healthy. Oh and the best part, get rid of the cancer that has interrupted your life. **Yes, you can!**

***

THE MIND-BODY CONNECTION

You cannot begin to heal, until you take control of your thoughts. Once the shock goes away and the "pity-party" stops, it's time to get your brain on board with your recovery. Many people are told, every day, that their cancer is terminal. Please, listen to me!!!! Only you decide when you are willing to give up. If you are ready to lay down and die, then you probably will. I know this sounds harsh, but I need to get through to you! You can choose life! Wake up every morning and commit yourself to learning about your cancer and the amazing things being done to treat it. There is a program out there just for you. Do your research and find the doctor that's right for your type of cancer. Arm yourself with the nutritional knowledge that you need. Remember the "Law of Attraction"? Make a vision board of your healthy self, doing the things you love, and *visualize* yourself healthy. Express your gratitude every day, for all the good things in your life, and stay active.

***

ENDINGS

It is not my time to die, this I know. It is, however, God's will for me to share my story of survival with others, hence this book. I will donate some proceeds from the book to two causes that are near and dear to me: "The National Breast Cancer Coalition" (www.breastcancerdeadline2020.org) and the "Make-A-Wish Foundation" (www.wish.org). We need more than "*hope*", we need a cure, and the coalition is the answer, in my opinion. Billions of dollars have been raised, in the name of "breast cancer," while the deaths from breast cancer remain virtually unchanged. I have plans on becoming an advocate for the NBCC. I am also a member of the "Michigan Breast Cancer Coalition" (www.mibcc.org). There are many other organizations that raise needed funds for breast cancer research.

I have made peace with death, since my mothers passing, after hearing what my mother had to say the day before she died. She said " My two little angels came to me and said that they are taking me home to heaven tomorrow. I am ready to go and I am not afraid". She sat up rather abruptly and appeared to be taking communion, although she was not catholic. She made the motion of drinking out of a goblet, using both hands, raising it to her lips, and tilting her head back to drink. She also was speaking to someone, and it clearly was not me. She was praying. She was so weak and I remember how startled I was when she sat up so abruptly. For months, she couldn't even lift her head! She did die the following day. I felt blessed that she had shared that moment with me. I was at peace when she died and knew that she was not alone, on her journey to heaven. But, with that said, I am not ready to die! Nor will I!

Just recently, I saw a link on Facebook, which led me to a book called "Revealing Heaven" by Kat Kerr. It is an amazing story of heaven and what life is like after death. If your cancer cannot be cured, or you know someone who has passed away from this terrible disease, please read that book. You will be transported to a place of peace and tranquility. Reading the book has been the perfect ending to my story, and hopefully "Revealing Heaven" will be the perfect beginning for much needed healing in this world!

**

RISK FACTORS

There are many known risk factors for breast cancer, including age, genetics, race, radiation, oral contraceptives, HRT, diet, alcohol, lack of exercise, insulin resistance, stress, inflammation, and EMF's. These by no means cover all of the causes. No matter what the cause of your cancer, know that blaming yourself will only make things worse. You must do everything now to cut your risk factors and reduce the spread of the cancer, in order to put it into remission. You will need to focus all of your energy on healing!

One very important risk factor is inflammation. So many things can cause havoc in our bodies, but inflammation is the one thing that you should be the most concerned about. Inflammation can be caused by our diets, stress, anger, depression, lack of physical activity, environmental pollution, and smoking. Cancer cells need inflammation to sustain their growth. Tumors use inflammatory substances to invade surrounding tissue, to go into the bloodstream, and to metastasize.

Everything we consume should be for our health. Our diets should be rich in Omega 3's. We should be on a ketogenic diet, eat organic food, and stay away from processed food, sugar, carbs, and dairy. We should get rid of the stress in our lives and exercise on a regular basis. We should get our insulin under control, get lots of oxygen (hyperbaric oxygen chamber) to prevent metastasis, and detox (infrared sauna). You must lose weight if you are obese and estrogen receptor positive (this will happen naturally with your new diet and exercise plan). We should laugh often and get rid of negative thoughts. You need to surround yourself with positive people and be positive. Get rid of any energy draining people in your life. You will need every weapon in your arsenal to beat cancer! Start today. All of this will reduce inflammation.

***

MY ANTI-CANCER DIET

Diet: Ketogenic

Breakfast:
Herbal decaf tea or decaf coffee
Heavy cream (1-2 teaspoons)
KetoCal shake 4:1 Ratio (**prescription**)
(Order from Nutricia North America)
30 g. of shake
Add 2 teaspoons of MCT oil (health food store)

Lunch:
3 cups of romaine, endive, or escarole,
or any dark leafy greens
Dressing made from lemon juice, coconut oil,
and water

Dinner:
1 cup of cooked broccoli (steamed)
or any green vegetable (non-starchy)
1 tablespoon coconut oil
Sardines in oil or 4 ozs. of protein

Snacks:

1 apple or 1 cup of strawberries
1 hard-boiled egg and 1 hard-boiled egg yolk
¼ of an avocado

SUPPLEMENTS, DRUGS, AND THERAPY

Supplements*

Digestive Enzymes:
10-15 minutes before each meal
Probiotics: 1 before breakfast
Wobenzym N:
3 twice a day on an empty stomach
(at least 45 minutes before meals)
Multigenics: (Metagenics)
1 with breakfast and 1 with dinner
Cal Apatite: (Metagenics) 1 with lunch
Mag Citrate: (Metagenics)
1 with lunch and 1 before bed
Vitamin D3: (Metagenics)
1 with breakfast and 1 with dinner
E400 Selenium: (Metagenics) 1 with dinner
Pleo Alkala Antacid Powder: (as per Dr.)
Super BioCurcumin: (LifeExtension)
1 with lunch and 1 before bed

(I order my supplements from:
www.naturalhealthyconcepts.com)
*Consult a nutritionalist
  Dosages will vary from person to person

Prescription Drugs
Celebrex
C-Naltrexone
Metformin HCL
Tamoxifen

**These drugs are specific to my case.
Each individual should consult a physician!**

Additional Therapy
Hyperbaric Oxygen Chamber (1.3-1.5 ATA)
3x per week for 1 hour to start
(reduce accordingly)

NUTRITIONAL SUPPLEMENTS

Curcumin: Antioxidant, anti-inflammatory, inhibitor of cancer, and protector of DNA. It blocks the cells that trigger inflammation, prohibiting the cancer to mutate. It promotes cell death, in cancer cells, without damaging other healthy cells.

Aloe Vera: Anti-inflammatory, immune stimulant, anti-cancer.

Selenium: Immune stimulant, reduces the toxicity of the chemo drug Adriamycin. Repairs DNA damage.

Enzymes: Taking Wobenzym, in between meals, can help to dissolve the coating around the cancer that makes it unseen by the immune system. Taking digestive enzymes before your meals can help to digest and absorb the food.

Vitamin D3: Attacks cancer at the genetic level

C-Naltrexone: Boosts the immune system, activating the body's own natural defenses. It stores the body's normal production of endorphins.

MCT Oil: It stands for Medium Chain Triglycerides. MCT's are naturally occurring in coconut and palm kernel oils. It is easily digested and rapidly metabolized for energy.

Virgin Coconut Oil: Coconut oil has anti-microbial properties, thus preventing the spread of cancer cells and enhancing the immune system. Virgin coconut oil is an effective anti-oxidant and prevents the formation of free radicals.

Lemon juice: Citrus flavonoids have anti-oxidant, anti-cancer, anti-viral, and anti-inflammatory effects.

Omega-3's: Reduces inflammation, reduces cancer growth, and reduces the spread of tumors.

CHANGES TO MAKE

- Avoid products containing chemicals, including cleaning and personal products.
- Eat grass fed organic animal products, in moderation.
- Increase your Omega-3 intake. (Sardines, mackerel, salmon, flax seed, nuts)
- Eat wild caught fish, not farm raised.
- Go on a ketogenic diet.
- Increase your intake of broccoli, brussel sprouts, cabbage, onion, leeks, and garlic, and citrus fruits.
- Eat an apple every day.
- Take supplements to stimulate your immune system and reduce inflammation.
- Filter water.
- Do not drink from plastic water bottles.
- Get 30 minutes of exercise a day.
- Relax and breathe. Do yoga, get a massage, and do deep breathing.
- Get oxygen. Start out with 3 days a week in the hyperbaric oxygen chamber. After 4 months you can probably reduce to 2 days a week.
- Detox (use an infrared sauna)
- Free yourself from negative emotions. Surround yourself with positive people, seek out therapy,

and do fun things that make you laugh. Make yourself and your health a priority.

- Cut out all sugar and sugar substitutes, except Stevia.
- Last, but not least (probably the most important thing) is find yourself a great doctor, who is on board with you! There are many holistic, alternative doctors out there!
- Do your research. There are many books available on cancer and nutrition.

IF I KNEW THEN, WHAT I KNOW NOW

- I wouldn't rush into surgery.
- I would have had a PET scan shortly after the mastectomy.
- I would have stressed less and laughed more.
- I would have researched alternative treatments earlier.
- I would have started to exercise sooner.
- I would have lost weight sooner.
- I would have kept working.
- I would have eaten healthier and read labels.
- I would have been more positive.
- I would have used more sunscreen.
- I would have gotten my hair cut really short before chemo.
- I would have given up bottled water.
- I wouldn't have eaten processed food & fast food.

MY FAVORITE THINGS

Doctors: Dr. Mark Rosenberg, M.D.
Dr. Linsey Gold, D.O. (Breast surgeon)
Dr. Kim Pummill, M.D. (Plastic surgeon)
Dr. Susan Longe, M.D.

Sports: Golf

Workout: Running

Running store:
Complete Runner, Flint, MI.

Wigs: *Katie's Spa*, Lapeer, MI.

Hair Stylist: Candy Holmes
Summerset Salon & Day Spa

Women's group: *UP Woman*

Organizations:
The Michigan Breast Cancer Coalition
The National Breast Cancer Coalition

Weight Loss Group: *Weight Watchers*

Sauna: Infrared sauna

Best for overall health:
Hyperbaric oxygen chamber
Dr. Benn, *Alternative Health & Rehab Centre*, Flint

Favorite workout aid: iPod

Favorite songs to run to:

Born This Way, Bad Romance (Lady Gaga)
What Doesn't Kill You, Makes You Stronger
(Kelly Clarkson)
Keep Pushin' (REO Speedwagon)

Athletic Club: *Davison Athletic Club*, Davison, MI.

Refresher drink:
The juice of 2 lemons, water, and Stevia.

Favorite charity: *Make–A-Wish Foundation*

SURVIVING CHEMOTHERAPY

1.   Prepare for chemo:
     Arrange for friends to take you, at least the first couple of times.
     Get a little cooler for snacks.
     Get a BPA free water bottle.
     Cut your hair short, and have wigs, hats, and scarves ready.
     Get a wig stand and wig shampoo.
     Get your nausea prescriptions filled.
     Get a book or magazines, or crossword puzzles, or whatever you enjoy doing.

2.   Stay out of the sun. Most likely, you will be on a drug that is light sensitive. Buy some long sleeve sun shirts, if you plan on being outside. Also, get some 100 SPF sunscreen.

3.   Eat healthy. Stay away from sugar. Remember that sugar FEEDS cancer!

4.   Walk and keep active.

5.   Get out and do things. (Go to the movies or lunch with friends)

6.   Let people help you. (One of the hardest things for me) People want to help. They are in this with you and are suffering, too. It also helps them to heal as well. They love you and want to be there for you, so let them! You will be glad you did! I could not have made it through chemo and cancer without the unwavering support of my husband, friends, and family! Give them suggestions on how they can help.

7.   Take biotin after chemo. It helps to grow strong hair and nails.

LEARNING TO RUN

When I decided to start running, to take the weight off, I couldn't even run for 15 seconds without feeling like I was going to die. Here is my beginning schedule for running:

Week 1: Run for 1 minute and walk for 9 minutes (total of ½ hour, 5 days a week)

Week 2: Run for 2 minutes and walk for 8 minutes (total of ½ hour, 5 days a week)

Week 3: Run for 3 minutes and walk for 7 minutes (total of ½ hour, 5 days a week)

Week 4: Run for 4 minutes and walk for 6 minutes (total of ½ hour, 5 days a week)

Week 5: Run for 5 minutes and walk for 5 minutes (total of ½ hour, 5 days a week)

Week 6: Run for 6 minutes and walk for 4 minutes (total of ½ hour, 5 days a week)

Week 7: Run for 7 minutes and walk for 3 minutes (total of ½ hour, 5 days a week)

Week 8: Run for 8 minutes and walk for 2 minutes (total of ½ hour, 5 days a week)

Week 9: Run for 9 minutes and walk for 1 minute (total of ½ hour, 5 days a week)

Gradually increase your workout time to 1 hour / 6 days a week.

When I run a long distance, like 10 miles, I run for 10 minutes and walk for 1 minute. You can do whatever is comfortable for you. I know some people who run for 1 minute and walk for 1 minute.

I run several 5K's and 8K's throughout the year, even in the winter, and my goal is to run a marathon.

ACKNOWLEDGMENTS

A sincere "thank you" to my husband Mark. I know you suffered though every minute as much as I did and I am sorry for the pain. Thanks to my many friends (you know who you are!) and my family, including my sister, Carol, for your support and prayers. Also, thanks to my doctors and their staff, for my treatments and surgeries. How do you really ever thank someone for saving your life? A special thank you to all my friends, at the Flint Elk's, who raised a huge amount of money for me, and are *always* there for me! Thank you to Candy for always making me look beautiful, and to Kim for the beautiful wigs and kind treatment! A special thank you to Kim and Rick for providing me with a year's worth of massages ….that was heavenly! Thank you to Steve Otte for the massages. Thank you to Tracey, Ken, and Mark for being my running buddies and to the people who inspired me to get into shape! Thank you to everyone who put me on their prayer lists and prayed for me, as I know that was a major factor in my recovery! Thank you to my dear friend, Pam Buerger, who sat through countless hours, with my husband, during my surgeries. Thank you for always being there for me! You are one in a million! A special thank you to my friends; Gail, Cheryl, and Kelley, who also suffered though breast cancer, around the same time as I did. Going through this journey with you three, made me feel as though I was *never* alone. Thank you to Mickey Cash (yes, related to Johnny Cash) for sharing your story of survival with me. You turned me in the right direction. You are an amazingly strong survivor of cancer, and a beautiful woman, inside and out, not to mention a very talented artist. Thank you to my graphic artists, Sheri Harvey, for my logos and Lori Tomlinson, for the book cover and web design. Thank you to Betty and Terry (bd's Mongolian Grill) for always supporting breast cancer causes. A special thank you to the women of "Up Woman" for making this book a reality. A big "thank you" to Suzanne Somers for the books that she put countless hours into researching, to help others. I was one that was helped tremendously by them! And last, but not least, thank you to my chemo buddies, Bill and Mark. Bill, you always knew just when to call, like you read my mind! You all have **amazing** strength and have helped me more than you will ever know! Thank you to everyone who has touched my life, in one way or another, during the past 4 years. There are too many people to mention, individually, but all have played a major role in my survival and recovery. I love you all!

***

Lori Baran is the author of *"After Cancer By Lori".* She was born in Dearborn, MI., and now resides in Atlas Township, MI. She is a graduate of Ferris State University, with a degree in Medical Laboratory Technology.

Her breast cancer was diagnosed in 2008. This book is her story of battling and conquering **Stage IV Metastatic Breast Cancer** with alternative methods.

www.aftercancerbylori

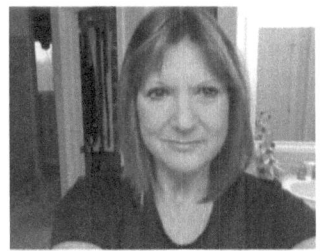